I0421878

My Unusual Stroke Story

Arianna Gabriel

Order this book online at www.trafford.com
or email orders@trafford.com

Most Trafford titles are also available at major online book retailers.

Printed in the United States of America.

ISBN: 978-1-4907-1477-6 (sc)
ISBN: 978-1-4907-1476-9 (e)

Trafford rev. 09/19/2013

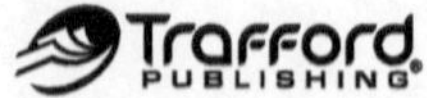

www.trafford.com

North America & international
tollfree: 1 888 232 4444 (USA & Canada)
fax: 812 355 4082

My Struggle to regain what was lost through
Prayer, Faith, and Humor

To my beloved husband, Vincent Lezama,
who has never left my side.
Without him my life would have been different.
And to my mother, who has passed away. She had three strokes.
Mom, I finally understand what you went through.

CONTENTS

PREFACE

Have faith and give thanks to God for even your smallest achievement.

Women have different physical symptoms than men in so many things. However, the symptoms of my stroke were very strange indeed.

My stroke caused me to have a temporary disability. That is what I say to myself. Although I do not have complete use of my right arm and leg, I consider that to be only temporary. I can walk with the use of a cane now, and I can use my right hand for some tasks. I have faith and have always projected a complete recovery. I always speak healing over my body, although I don't see the immediate healing like you see on TV. Still, I have never doubted my healing.

In my dreams I am always going about doing my chores and running errands in a complete state. I have never seen myself as disabled. Thank God strokes can be treated and prevented, as long as you keep your blood pressure, cholesterol, and blood sugar under control. Always visit your doctor to get them checked.

After my stroke I was completely paralyzed on the right side of my body. I had no control of the muscles on the right side of my face or my right arm and leg. This caused me great difficulty with walking, eating, and dressing. When I did physical therapy, I started to see slight improvement in muscle movement.

Weeks after I had the stroke, I became sensitive to the cold on the affected side, but that is gradually improving now. My husband's niece suggested I join a recreational center to do water exercises, so I became a member and started swimming a few days a week. I say that loosely because I cannot swim. Many of the other members would say to me, "I can't believe you are from the Caribbean and you cannot swim." I put on so many floatation devices, all I did was spin around in the water like a top.

The other women in the class constantly had to turn me around. They had a good laugh at me, but it was fun. I was convinced that water therapy was the way to go. I took the classes for a few months, thoroughly enjoying them because they had me laughing and my favorite instructor, Kathy, was very funny. I always enjoyed any class she instructed. I was unable to continue, though, because my right side was always freezing from the coldness of the water. Although I love the water, I just could not get warm in that pool.

My doctor gave me various medications, but nothing helped. All they did was leave me completely incapacitated. On one occasion he prescribed a very strong painkiller. Well, I was so high and sleeping for days, it became impossible for me to function. I had absolutely no quality of life from being high on those pills. I hated the way they made me felt, and I stopped before I became addicted.

I started to withdraw from my family and friends, becoming antisocial, because they did not seem to understand that I was unable to do certain things. They would ask why I didn't do something or why I didn't want to go somewhere with them. I wanted to shout at them, "Because I cannot do those things you want me to do."

So I stayed away from them. If I was not feeling well, I would only tell my husband or my closest friend, Maude. They really encouraged me to do what I was comfortable doing.

Vince is my champion. He only saw my achievements, not my failures. He would say, "Next time you will do it." Although I might have been down, I always took great care of myself with the help of my husband and Maude. One thing I strongly suggest if you've had a stroke is to make sure you are out of bed and dressed. This will make you feel better. If you are unable to move, ask someone to put you in a chair if it is allowed by your doctor. This really is good for you. Get out of those nightclothes.

Maintain your selfesteem, stay connected, and be interested in what is going on in the world. Although the news can be dreary at times, pay attention. If you can understand what is going on, you are on the road to recovery.

My stroke was a lifechanging event for me. It affected my emotions. At times I felt frustrated, but that was not the way to go. I had to maintain my positive mood. My husband kept me laughing, but as I had no control of my bladder, there were lots of accidents. He didn't mind washing all those wet undergarments. I thank God for him every day.

One of the downsides of having a stroke is a diminished sex drive. I was in so much pain, Vince felt sorry for me and left me alone.

These are some of the things I've learned. They will be important for your recovery:

Do not be hard on yourself. Only with time, physical therapy, occupational therapy, and hard work will you see results.

Do not shut yourself away. Get out of the house. Go to the recreational center if there is one in your neighborhood. Go to a restaurant for a meal if you can. Do not be selfconscious around others when eating. Just thank God you can do it. If you are bedridden, ask your caregiver to get you up in a chair and place it near a window. Seeing the activity outside can lift your spirits. Do not get discouraged. Thank God for what you can do. Remember, getting out of the house is good for you. That is therapy.

Join a support group. It is helpful to meet other stroke patients who are struggling with the same problems as you, share your experiences, and make new friends. Have a phone conversation at least once a day. Just call someone. It will help you feel connected with friends and family, which will start to make you feel confident. If you are unable to communicate, try using cue cards. You will find them very helpful. Also, appreciate even the smallest things in life. Do not focus on what you cannot do.

Always stay positive and have lots of laughter. First thing in the morning I thank God for keeping me through the night and waking me up. I surround myself with laughter. I will call my friend Jackie, and after some jokes we will laugh so long and hard, anything that was bothering us will suddenly seem inconsequential. One day I was having lunch and wanted my husband to get me something. It was very frustrating because I could not pronounce the word. Needless to say, my husband and I started laughing.

See yourself as completely healed, believe it, and it is done. Record your progress, and celebrate every milestone you make. Always keep God first in everything you do, and give him thanks. I have learned that whenever my faith seems to be at its lowest, I cast out that spirit of fear and take back control. Most of all, *say it with authority.*

ACKNOWLEDGMENTS

Thanks to my children Andine, Jillian, Georgina, and my soninlaw Jay for their endless support.

To my grandchildren Cheyenne, Tsashai, Daveana, Gabriel, and Gianna. I love you all.

Thanks to Maude for being a good friend and giving me endless moral support.

To my sister Catherine for all her prayers and moral support.

Also to my aide Maria Newell. You are called to heal and be a blessing to others.

To Dianne in Trinidad, who calls me repeatedly to pray for me.

To Gail for all the encouragement and advice she gave me.

Also to Jackie for being a good friend and confidante who was always there for me.

INTRODUCTION

I was looking forward to my vacation. My husband and I were going on a cruise, and one of the stops was Jamaica. The cruise was everything I desired. We had a room with a balcony where I was able to have some quiet time and read my book. The peaceful ocean had a calming effect on me as I daydreamed. On this particular cruise I saw a rainbow on the water. I wished for a pot of gold, but that was only fantasy. *Ah!* I thought, staring at the water. *What a life.*

I had a wonderful time in all of the islands we visited. Each one had its unique quality and activities, but Jamaica was the best for me as I climbed the famous Dunn's River Falls. The guide divided us into separate groups, and we sang the chorus our guide taught us. My husband did not enjoy climbing the falls because he was cold in the river water, but it was great for me. That water kept me cool in the heat. I thoroughly enjoyed being in the tropics. After climbing the falls, we did some sightseeing and sampled some of those wonderful Jamaican dishes.

After having so much fun on my trip, I took another week vacation to recover from my vacation. I could never go on vacation and then directly return to work. It takes too much out of me. I have to take a week to rest because I really exert myself whenever I am away, and this time was no different. So during that second week I started to prepare myself to return to work. On the Saturday before I returned to my job, I went out shopping to get myself some new clothes. I had a new slimmeddown body that I was proud of and eager to show off.

As I visited various stores, I started to have extreme pain all over my back. I was not feeling well, but as I had recently lost fiftytwo pounds, I made that my motivation to keep on shopping. Also, there was a beautiful Calvin Klein coat calling my name, and being humble as I was, I just had to answer. It looked so good on me I thought I was a model. Also, I was looking forward to returning to the office so I could tell my colleagues about my vacation and show them the many, many pictures I took.

That night the awful pain lodged in my upper back. It was a strange pain; I usually suffer from lower back pain, and this was much worse. I asked my husband to rub my back with an ointment I had in the medicine cabinet. I said to him, "This is the worst pain I have ever had. The last time I had such awful pain, there was a little person in a cot nearby to show for it." That night I hardly slept.

The next day was Sunday, and no matter how I felt, I knew that I was going to my job the next day. I was definitely not calling in sick. It was not going to look good to call in after my vacation.

As a human resources manager, I frequently had to reprimand employees for calling in the day after their vacation, so I definitely had to suck it up and go to work. Many times I have wondered if the blood clot was in my lungs and then traveled to my brain, if that is even possible. I will never know as I am not a doctor, and I never remembered to mention it to them.

CHAPTER 1

The Day I had Strange Symptoms That Turned Out to Be an Unusual Stroke.

Monday morning arrived. The air smelled fresh as I woke up bright and early and happily got ready for work. Vince had my breakfast ready for me as usual. I always have it in the car on Mondays during our long trip from Bethlehem, Pennsylvania, to Queens, New York. Though we lived in Bethlehem, we had an apartment in Queens where we stayed during the week while I worked. After eating my breakfast in the car, I usually took a nap. I said goodbye to him as he dropped me off at the nursing home where I worked.

I had arrived early, and everyone was excited to see me. "Miss Yvonne is back," they all said, surrounding me. The employees were asking me so many questions, I just had to make the rounds, describing my vacation and showing everyone my pictures. I still was not feeling well, and my body was aching all over again. I took two painkillers.

I finally decided it was time I settled down to work. After all, I was getting good pay for a day's work. However, all through the morning I was in agony. I took more painkillers and wondered what was really going on with my body. I had a doctor's appointment for the next evening but was seriously thinking of calling his receptionist to see if I could reschedule for that day.

At one o'clock, while having lunch in the director's office, I said to her, "The only way I can finish the day is to keep taking painkillers. Something is really wrong with my body." I was still feeling awful and had so much pain. She thought I might be coming down with the flu, saying she had felt the same over the weekend and suggesting I go home. Considering the way I felt, I was desperate to take her advice, but I stuck it out instead and left at the usual time.

The Day I Had Strange Symptoms That Turned Out to Be an Unusual Stroke

The next day were Tuesday November 1, 2011—another beautiful day, the first of the month, and the day before my birthday. The air was crisp, and it felt so good. I love fall. The way the air felt, I wondered about the winter that was coming. Would it be mild or harsh? I love winter too. I love the snow and cannot wait for it to get here. Many people think I am crazy and make comments like, "You are from the Caribbean and you don't like heat?" Regardless, I was really looking forward to the next day since it was my birthday and I would be spending the evening with my husband, Vince, at his favorite restaurant.

For a few days he had been talking about going to City Island for a lobster and crab dinner. He loves to go to Sammy's restaurant, he loves crab legs and lobster tails, and he particularly loves the huge portions they serve because he can have the leftovers the next day. Although I tell him about the high cholesterol seafood contains, he ignores me.

I woke up Tuesday still feeling a bit off. I was lightheaded, but my body was not aching anymore. I knew something was still wrong, although I could not put my finger on the exact problem.

If someone had asked me to give him an exact description of my feelings, I would not have been able to. All I could say was that I was feeling very strange. So I told myself to suck it up. I wasn't a baby, and I would get through the day just fine. Showering and dressing, however, were taxing. I had to try hard to get it done. Why was I feeling like this? I couldn't say specifically what was happening to me. I was not weak, and I did not have any aches. So I put on my makeup, ate my breakfast, and went out the door.

I had to get to work by seven thirty, so I left my New York apartment and drove to work as usual, not knowing this would be the last time for a long time that I'd be able to do these things I'd taken for granted. While sitting in my office, I had the same uncomfortable feeling that I couldn't describe.

I decided to visit the nurse who worked on the first floor of the nursing home. Mrs. Patel is a lovely nurse, very caring and thorough. I felt guilty interrupting her while she was attending to the residents, but today was significantly different. She didn't seem to mind the interruption. She took my blood pressure and measured my blood sugar, and then she reassured me that everything was normal.

On my way back to the office I met many employees who complimented me on my outfit, stating that I looked great. I laughed and modeled my outfit, not wanting them to know that anything was wrong. I was enjoying the attention because it had been years since I was this size.

I knew the others would make a fuss if they knew I didn't feel well, and that was the last thing I wanted. I could not wait to get back to my office so that I could sit down, but for some reason that walk to the office seemed longer than usual. When I sat at my desk, I mentioned to my coworker, Fran, that I thought I might be having a stroke. She replied, "You don't have any symptoms of a stroke."

I agreed but then said that women have different symptoms than men in so many ailments. I then remembered the burning sensation I'd had in my left eye over the weekend. I told her about it and that awful upper back pain I'd had and that I'd still had the pain that day before and had taken painkillers all day.

My left eye had had that same burning sensation when I woke up that morning, as though someone had thrown hot sauce in my eye. Fran said that still wasn't a symptom of a stroke. Well! Everyone in the office knew that if you were feeling ill, all you had to do was tell Fran your symptoms and she'd give you an accurate diagnosis. She had wanted to be a doctor, but due to circumstances out of her control, she did not fulfill her dream. She would have been a very good doctor.

So when she said I was not having the symptoms of a stroke, I believed her. As it turned out, even the doctors in the emergency room agreed with her. A stroke occurs when the blood supply to your brain is severely reduced, preventing the brain from getting oxygen. However, as I learned later, my brain was getting good oxygen. I knew that having a stroke is an emergency. Immediate action should be taken to minimize brain damage, but I did not have any symptoms. Stroke symptoms are very clear.

- Weakness of the limbs so that you have difficulty walking. You may stumble and lose your balance, have no coordination, or get very dizzy.
- Slurred speech and difficulty in speaking. You may also be unable to understand what is been said.
- Blurry vision. Your eyes may become blurry, or you might have double vision.
- Drooping of the face.

I had none of the above, although I was feeling a little unsteady. I thought everything was going to be all right, so I decided to start recording some appointments in the consultants' book so the consultants might be able to see the residents that day.

As I started to write, I saw that I couldn't make the number four. No matter how I tried, it looked like chicken scratch. I decided to call my doctor. It was time. I had an appointment with him that evening, but I wanted to see if I could change the appointment time so I could see him immediately.

After hearing my voice over the phone—I didn't know he was hearing slurred speech; to me I sounded normal—he told me to go to the emergency room immediately. My coworkers wanted to call an ambulance, but I wouldn't hear of it. I had too much pride to be taken out in an ambulance of all things. It would be so embarrassing.

Furthermore, I looked too good in my new outfit to be carted off in an ambulance, so I called my husband to come and take me to the emergency room. The hospital was about fifteen minutes away from the nursing home, but my apartment was literally only two minutes away. He took forever, so I called him a second time, asking him to come now. He told me later that he heard the urgency in my voice when I called the second time and became very concerned.

Apparently, when I had called before, he was just about to get into the shower. He did not think it was as serious as a stroke. Furthermore, I had only left about an hour earlier looking fine, so what could have gone wrong in such a short time? I had not said anything to him that morning about how I was feeling.

When he arrived, everyone wanted to help me get to the car, but that darn pride again made me say no. I was going to do it on my own, even though I was very unsteady by then. On our way to the hospital, I told Vince that my doctor was the one who'd suggested I go to the emergency room immediately. Vince put his foot down on the gas pedal and broke every speed limit on the way.

We kept talking. He did not seem to notice the slurring of my speech or just did not want to mention it to me. He drove to the ambulance section of the emergency room and came around to help me out of the car. I did it on my own, so he got me a wheelchair and took me inside.

When we arrived in the waiting room, a clerk asked me for my medical card and a few other questions, and then she handed me some papers to sign. I took the pen from her, and it was then I realized I was unable to write anything. My fingers could not even grip the pen. They immediately rushed me into the triage area and called on the overhead speakers for a stroke team STAT.

A neurologist and his team came in and gave me numerous tests. He told me to touch his finger with my left index finger. That was fine. However, when he gave me the same instruction and told me to use my right index finger, everything changed. I could not even lift my hand much less touch his finger. He said that it looked like a stroke, but he could not give me the drug tPA (which can break up a blood clot and stop the stroke from progressing) because he did not know if the stroke had started during the night. Three hours could have passed already.

He explained to me that the drug had to be administered within three hours of a stroke beginning; otherwise, I could have bleeding in the brain. He sent me for an MRI. It was around 8:30 or 9:00 a.m. at that time. After that I had a CT scan. I spent all day in the emergency room just lying there watching many people come and go. Needless to say, I got restless. All I could think about was that the next day was my birthday, the big 60. Was this the way it was going to start?

The nurses started an IV drip of heparin, and I tried not to think about what was going on. Strangely enough, I was not scared or panicking. I felt very calm and serene, as if this was not happening to me. I knew everything was going to be all right. I told myself I was just lying there and soon I would be able to get up and leave. Or so I thought. During my stay in the emergency room, the nurses took thirteen vials of blood from me. I felt like a regular pincushion.

It suddenly hit me that every ten years something happened to me. When I was forty, all I wanted was to have sex. There were times when I seriously thought of going to the doctor, but it subsided. Then at fifty I started to wet the bed for no apparent reason. I did go to the doctor for that. He gave me a medication, and it stopped. And now at sixty it was a stroke. I wondered what was going to happen when I am seventy. I decided not to claim any tenyear pattern. I had to put a stop to that, linking what was taking place every ten years in my body. I declared that seventy would come without incident.

Meanwhile everyone was going about his or her business, no one was explaining anything to me, and I was starving. I needed something to eat and asked a nurse to please give me some lunch. I saw some of the patients eating, and I was so hungry. The nurse told me that the doctor would have to approve it. I waited, but no food appeared. When I finally saw the doctor hours later, I pleaded with him to please approve an order for me to get something to eat. He said he would and left the area. Needless to say, that was the last time I saw him.

As I lay in the emergency room, I reflected on my life and had the urge to talk with someone. I called my sister Catherine, even though I was not supposed to use my cell phone, and tried to explain to her where I was and that I had suffered a stroke that morning. For some reason she kept asking me what I'd just said. In my head it sounded good, I was speaking perfect English. Why didn't she understand? I repeated myself so many times, I was getting frustrated.

Apparently when she could not understand what I was saying, she realized I'd had a stroke and started to cry. That made me cry also, but why was she crying? Maybe it was worse than I thought. I looked at my husband, puzzled. He took the phone away from me and spoke with Catherine, explaining what had happened and giving her a progress report. The conversation was brief because he did not want to upset me. Still he had not told me that my speech was affected so badly, it was difficult for anyone to understand me.

Around nine that night the nurses came to take me for another CT scan. I did not know why I had to have another one.

After the scan I was told that there was an available room on the fifth floor. It was after nine thirty when I was taken to a room with the heparin drip in my arm. When I got upstairs, Maria Newell, the nursing assistant assigned to my room, got me settled into bed. She was very thorough and got me all tucked in before she left. That night was really rough for me. The drip in my arm was painful, I was unable move, and I needed to go to the bathroom regularly, so all night I kept ringing the bell. I felt sorry for putting anyone through that. I do not like to be a problem to others, but it was unavoidable,

Thank God the person who came regularly was Maria. She was very patient and kind to me, especially when she had to roll me from side to side. I kept apologizing because I felt guilty for bothering her all night. Early the next morning the phlebotomist came for another eleven vials of blood. I asked her what they were doing with all that blood, although I knew they had to do various tests. I also told her, should anything accidentally slip out of my mouth, not to take it personally, because I was bad with needles. Then I just relaxed as best as I could and let her get on with it. Soon after that Maria came in to make sure I was comfortable and clean before she left to go home. I was very grateful.

CHAPTER 2

A Caribbean custom is to keep a nutmeg in your mouth to prevent drooping caused by a stroke. Also, we use it if we think a stroke is coming on or if we've already had a stroke. So that morning I asked my niece Nekeisha to go to the grocery store and get me some nutmegs. She brought me a bag of nutmegs.

Later that day I realized I did not have to ask her to make a special trip to the store. It seemed like every Caribbean visitor who came to see me brought nutmegs. It did not matter which island they came from, they all knew about it. To use the nutmeg, you crack the shell and put the whole nutmeg in your mouth. Some even brought me a mixture of grated nutmeg and various oils to rub on my affected limbs.

Someone wanted to know if he could use the nutmeg powder in his mouth instead. I told him no. You could only mix the powder with various oils to rub on your limbs. All of these remedies came from our parents and grandparents. (Under no circumstances am I suggesting that anyone do the same if it is not your custom. I am not a doctor, and I am too old for prison. Someone my age should be coming out, not going in.) I am only saying that it is a Caribbean custom that the nutmeg prevents your mouth from drooping; or if it has already drooped, it corrects it. I grew up seeing stroke patients with nutmegs in their mouths. If someone had a severe headache and didn't knowing what was causing it, most likely an older person gave him a nutmeg to put in his mouth while seeking medical attention.

Later that day the hospital was inundated with the staff from the nursing home where I worked. The eveningshift employees came before going to work—their shift started at 3:30 p.m.—and the dayshift employees came after 3:30 p.m. when their shift ended. The nightshift workers came after their shift ended in the morning.

On my birthday, November 2, I turned sixty years old and almost did not see the day. I thanked God for waking me up that morning. I always thank him for waking me. It is a practice I've done since I was young, but that day it really had a different meaning to me. *I was alive.*

That day my friend and coworker Maude came to visit me on her lunch break. She immediately started massaging my right arm and leg, checking my range of motion. (Of all my coworkers, she was one of the few who was not constantly crying and was determined to lift my spirits.) She did rangeofmotion exercises each time she visited, and then she came back in the evening to wash me and make sure I was clean and comfortable.

She did that for my entire nineday stay at the hospital. I was lucky to have a friend like her. I felt so guilty because she was working so hard on my limbs. She was shorter than me, and God alone knows how she managed, since I was dead weight. Although I strongly protested, telling her she didn't have to do this, she completely ignored me.

Maude told me that the staff at the Cliffside Nursing Home had planned a surprise birthday party for me, so everything at the nursing home was now in disarray. Many of the employees had prepared dishes from their different countries and brought them to work, not realizing I was in the hospital with a stroke.

Maude had been on vacation when I was. She was still in Florida on November 1 but planned on coming back that night since she was the organizer of the party. She was preparing some of the dishes too. She cooked at her daughter's house in Florida and brought the food back with her on her flight to New York. I really cannot imagine how she did that.

She said as soon as the plane landed, she got many calls from the staff who were at work that day when I got ill, informing her of my condition and not knowing what to do about the party. They had no option but to go ahead with the party. I was told it was very somber.

The next day Maude brought a huge cake to the hospital and took lots of pictures of me holding it, together with two huge cards that had many signatures from the staff. It was lovely. All the nurses in the hospital wished me happy birthday. It was not what I had envisioned for my birthday, but thank God I could enjoy the cake and be happy I was alive. I said to myself, *Where there is life, there is hope. I am alive, so I hope to be out of this bed very soon.*

Maude shared the cake with the nurses and my roommate at the hospital. Flowers were being delivered by the hour from family and friends, as well as the doctors, administrators, and my coworkers at the nursing home. It made me feel loved and appreciated. Meanwhile, my husband, Vince, was feeling all alone but trying his best not to show me how concerned he was.

That evening, one of my coworkers went to the airport to pick up a Sevenday Adventist pastor from Jamaica who was on vacation in this country. Instead of taking him to his destination, she brought him to see me at the hospital so that he could pray for me.

I really appreciated that. Then my sister Catherine came with my nephew Brendan and her good friend Shirley. Everyone started crying, and so did I. That evening my stepdaughter Lisa and her husband, Doug, were also at my bedside. I was very happy to see them.

My sister started to pray, and everyone participated. That felt good. They were all praying with me. I also received international calls from evangelists' friends and relatives, all praying for me over the phone. When a cousin of mine in Trinidad heard I had had a stroke, she and her two sisters started a novena for me by going to nine churches that day. I had never had so many people praying for me before, and it felt so good.

I have always tried to do something good for people, and I am always ready to help anyone who needs it. A nursing assistant at the nursing home suddenly died in her apartment and was going to be buried in a potter's field. That did not feel right to me, so I took it upon myself to start begging everyone for donations, and boy, did I *beg*.

The funeral director was speechless when I came up with the money, and she had a beautiful funeral with a massive turnout from the staff. These are the things I like to do, not for recognition but because it feels good. So now I was receiving the blessings, and it felt good. After everyone had left, my favorite nursing assistant came to my room, and as usual I was looking forward to seeing her. As she took care of me, she would massage my weak limbs and constantly pray under her breath, not knowing that I was listening.

Maria reassured me that I would get better. God had healed her from a similar situation. Her condition had been worse than mine—she was unable to speak—so he would definitely heal me. She was a devout Sevenday Adventist. If I had had any doubts before about my recovery, which I had not, they went out the window. At that time my faith got stronger. I had no doubt I was already healed. You have to learn not to pay attention to the symptoms. I knew that I was already healed. It did not matter that I couldn't move. I was a true believer.

Many of the nurses told me stories of their recoveries from severe ailments—how they had been healed—and they gave all the praise and thanks to God. My sisterinlaw, Vince's sister, and her daughter Loraine came, and I felt accepted by the family. Vince and I had been married for only two years.

That day I sent an email to my husband's niece Diane in Trinidad. (I was able to use my iPad by typing with my left index finger.) When Diane received the email, she was not sure where it had come from and who had sent it. She called the number I included in the email to find out if it was a wrong message or a message intended for someone else.

When I spoke with Diane, she also could not understand me. It took her awhile to realize what I was saying, and then she recognized that it was her uncle's wife who she had called. After that she gave me some encouraging words and told me I was going to be fine. She started to pray for my recovery and my complete healing—*in Jesus's name*. She is what we call a praying mantis, also known as a prayer warrior.

She prayed with me for about twenty minutes, and all the time I felt as though something was going through my body. I am not sure if it was my imagination, but I was very sure about this—I saw myself just getting up and walking out. I am not religious, I do not go to church, but I know for a fact nothing is impossible with the Lord. I was taught to ask for anything in Jesus's name, believe I would receive it, and then thank him, for it is done. From that time I have thanked him for his mercy and my healing. Also, my name is Lord, so I know that I have my own private line.

My daughter Andine, who is in the United States Army, was in Iraq at the time. My other daughters—Jillian, who lives in Maryland, and Georgina, who lives in Virginia—were all anxious about my prognosis. They were preparing themselves for the trip to New York. However, my husband advised them to be calm and wait until they heard from him because I was doing well. We all knew Andine would have been unable to come see me, but her sisters were keeping her updated on the situation.

Bernadette, my brother's wife and also an employee of Cliffside, and Joan, a close family friend, came to see me the day after my birthday after working the night shift. That was a very traumatic visit. We were all wailing so hard. They were holding on to me, very upset at seeing me in that position. The wailing went on for a while, their tears falling on my forehead, face, and chest like raindrops. When we were finished with all that crying, we looked at each other and started laughing and talking.

We really had a lovely visit. The only downside was that I was in the bed, unable to move. As usual, Maude was there twice a day fussing around, making sure I had what I needed. She asked me if the doctor had told the nurses to get me out of bed yet. When I told her no, she said, "I am getting you out of bed and into a chair because if you don't get up, recovery will be much harder." I wondered how she was going to accomplish that on her own, but she did.

She struggled to get me into the chair, and then she propped me up with pillows to support me. Since my right side was weak, I was leaning to the right. One thing I discovered was that it's important to start ambulating as soon as possible when you have a stroke. Maude's job at the nursing home is to ambulate the residents and to do rangeofmotion exercises with them, so she knew what had to be done.

One of the nursing assistants at the nursing home came to visit and brought me some documents. One of them was a family leave paper from work that needed a doctor's signature. This document had to be returned to my employer as soon as possible. I told the assistant I would give it to the doctor the next day and then return it to the facility with one of the employees visiting me. I knew the payroll department needed it.

As usual, that evening my room was very crowded. I was told that they had stopped counting the many, many visitors who came to my room. At one point the security officer at the front desk wanted to know the name of the VIP they were visiting. I had never been called that before.

One nursing assistant said to me that they would miss my husband's cooking. Many times he will get up around 4:00 a.m. to make one of his famous Caribbean breakfasts, which I would take to the facility for the office staff. Vince just loves to cook and see people enjoy the meals he creates in the kitchen, which is why the doctor had to put me on a diet. The nursing director once said that my husband was fattening me so that no one would look at me. We had a good laugh over that.

A friend of mine from Philadelphia called her daughter Dianne, who lived in New York, and asked her to come to the hospital to see me, which she did. Two days later a man I didn't recognize came to my room asking if I needed anything. I said no and thanked him, but then I asked who he was. He told me he was a security guard at the hospital and his friend Dianne had told him to check in on me every day while he was at work and to get me anything I needed. I was humbled. He checked in on me for the rest of my stay.

Many people sent flowers and plants to me, so my bedside table was very crowded. My coworkers continued to visit, and all the doctors who visited the nursing home came to the hospital to see me. Now I know that they really appreciated what I did for them.

The team of doctors that was attending to me was doing everything possible. I was told I had a wonderful team, but the doctors were unsure of how to classify my symptoms. There was no bleeding in my brain, and they still did not see a blood clot. I asked them what they were treating if they did not know if it was a stroke. They told me there were no different treatments for strokes; they only treated with things like heparin, and I was also getting aspirin. That did not reassure me because here I was, paralyzed on the right side and unable to speak properly, and all they could say was that I had strokelike symptoms.

I gave the doctor my family leave paper for his signature. When he brought it back the next day, he told me he could only affirm that I had strokelike symptoms until there was definite proof of a stroke. Still, he was treating me as he would any other stroke patient.

That evening the nursing assistant from my job who had brought the visiting pastor from Jamaica returned. She brought her entire prayer group from her church with her, including her grandson. About twelve to fifteen people were there, and they had a complete church service around my bed. Lots of singing and preaching went on and I thoroughly enjoyed it, but it was really getting loud and I worried about my roommate in the next bed. However, she shouted that she needed some of those prayers. The service lasted fifteen to twenty minutes. I felt the blessing, and after that I felt as though I was on cloud nine and ready to welcome my many, many visitors that evening.

Although I couldn't move, never at any time did I feel sorry for myself. I had learned from my mother never to say *Why me?* but *Why not me?* Why should it be someone else? What made me more special than anyone else?

CHAPTER 3

I would not wish a stroke on anyone. I just want to thank all the staff at Cliffside Nursing Home for their compassion, prayers, and concern. From the administrator to the kitchen aide, they all lifted my spirits. Also, I thanked God that I was alive, although I was unable to move. Many stroke patients are unable to respond and are unaware of their surroundings. I was in a good place, thank God.

The fourth day went by as usual, with the same amount of visitors coming all day long. I was rarely alone, and when I was, Maria was there, checking in on me and giving me words of encouragement. Maude was often there to make sure I was comfortable. My husband would always have me laughing—he should have been a comedian—and laughter is a very good medicine. It puts you in a positive mood, which keeps you from obsessing over a bad situation.

I am not saying you won't feel depressed if you have a stroke, but as soon as that happens, cast it out of you. I knew it was a done deal with the Lord. If you do not believe in Jesus, pray to whomever you pray to. I did not have to focus on my physical body, only on my spiritual. It is difficult to explain, but it was as if I only had a headache and I was able to keep my same happy personality.

The nurses and my friends turned me from side to side whenever necessary—I felt like a sack of potatoes being tossed around—but to me that was not a problem. The only time I was uncomfortable was when my friend Maude saw me naked. After working with her for more than ten years, I felt exposed. I tried to cover my nakedness at first, but I soon got over the embarrassment. I realized that this is life. You could be in the best of health in the morning and by the evening, disaster could strike.

On many occasions Mrs. Patel, the nurse who had taken my vital signs the morning when I had the unusual Stroke symptoms at the nursing home, would bring me supper, preparing her Indian dishes for me. If she was unable to visit, she would send it with her daughter. I always looked forward to seeing that meal.

You just have to appreciate life and what you have. I praise God every minute of the day. I talk to him constantly. As I said before, I am not religious, but I firmly believe in my God. I don't go to church, but I have been in the process of finding one now. I like the churches that are lively and where I feel comfortable. I would watch Joel Osteen on television and go to his meetings whenever he was in my state.

Before, I was always too busy to pray, always making excuses. I was tired, not realizing that you don't have to say anything special. I had always thought you have to be so fluent with your prayer and be able to go on praying for a while, but then I learned you just talk to God like you are talking to a friend. If you have a problem, just give it to him.

Many years ago I wondered how a person gives God her problems. That concept was difficult for me to digest. I did not understand, but as soon as I understood the concept of giving God the problems that I couldn't solve, it became very simple. I soon learned to believe and have faith. Now that is a done deal. I always give my problems to the Lord and don't worry about them anymore. Then I thank him for the solutions.

On Saturday, November 5, the fifth day of my stay at the hospital, the doctor ordered another MRI. This time he said it would be of the back of my head and neck. The orderly came to transport me to the MRI room as soon as some of my visitors arrived. I was surprised because I hadn't expected them to come to New York, but they told me not to worry myself. They would be right there when I got back. So the orderly took me downstairs for my second MRI.

The technician who did the MRI assured me that the doctor would get the results that same day.

"Finally," I said, "he will know once and for all what gave me that stroke."

After the second MRI was done, the orderly brought me back to my room where my visitors were waiting. My team of doctors came around to see me that evening and said they had found a blood clot in my brain stem.

"Imagine that," I said. "I have never heard that it takes five days in the hospital to discover you have a blood clot in your brain after giving the patient one MRI and two CT scans. This must be a record. Why didn't you order a complete MRI before, one that also scanned my neck?"

One of the doctors explained that it was the worst place to have a blood clot.

"Great," I said. "That really reassures me." But again, I knew I was covered. All those prayers went up, and the blessings came down. I just kept saying, "Thank God. I am blessed."

The doctor tried to explain what had happened in a simple way. The brain stem is the junction box that controls everything. It is the main computer that controls speech, movements, and everything else. Again I said that was not reassuring. I asked him to make sure to send the report to my family doctor. I heard later from my doctor that the report shocked him and made him very upset. A few weeks earlier, before my vacation, he had ordered a blood workup for me, and everything was good. He said to me, "You were not a candidate for a stroke. All your numbers were good."

All I could think of was to thank God that they had finally found the cause of the stroke and now it was rehabilitation time. That evening when my husband came to see me, I gave him the news, and we both looked forward to the next step toward my recovery. That weekend I had the usual visitors. There were the usual prayers and laughter, but I was eagerly looking forward to seeing the doctors on Monday.

Ah! Monday arrived, and I was waiting patiently for the doctors to make their rounds, wondering what they were going to do about me. Every other time they came around, they just stared at me and took notes, and then they ordered more blood work. Today they knew I had a blood clot, so I needed answers from the doctors and was eager for them to do something differently. The doctor had ordered physical therapy for me on my second day at the hospital. The physical therapist came on the fourth day with a walker, not knowing that I couldn't even turn myself in bed much less walk. He was unprepared and not properly equipped.

I couldn't imagine what the doctor's order might have been. *This is incompetence*, I thought. Had the doctor given the physical therapist the wrong orders, or did the physical therapist just assume I could use a walker? Thank God he was not my therapist, because his attitude was less than desirable. As far as I know, the doctors hadn't ordered the nurses to get me out of bed. It was my friend Maude who decided it was time to prop me up in a chair.

When my husband came in on Monday, he informed me that he would try to get me walking. *What?* I couldn't stand, I told him. Had he missed that from all his visits?

"I know," he said, laughing at the expression of fright on my face. "Please trust me."

Well, there is trust and there is *trust*. Hesitantly I said, "Try, but please, do not let me end up on the floor." He struggled to get me to the edge of the bed, but eventually he did. I was thinking, *What a brave man*. What was he thinking? What did he have for breakfast that morning? Also, the man is so skinny—over seventy years old, but he looks fifty—and he wanted to do this alone.

I believe the man found the fountain of youth. He loves it when people discover his true age, because they gasp in disbelief and ask others if they believe this man is over seventy. With a proud smile on his face he whips out his driver's license. It is like showandtell.

Finally, he lifted me to stand up, but my right foot kept sliding all over the place. I had no support from it. That was a sight to behold, but he did it. He held me very, very tight around my waist and literally dragged me a few steps.

That was exhausting. The whole room was spinning so fast, and I was screaming, "Please, I am going to fall." He dragged me back to bed, totally supporting my dead weight. Was that love? I wondered. All I know is that was very difficult for him.

Later on that day the doctor came to my room. Since we knew the blood clot was in my brain stem, he could now speak with the social worker to arrange a rehabilitation facility for me. Hopefully I would be discharged the next day.

The social worker came to see me that evening, asking if I had a preference of rehabilitation hospitals. I told her I wanted to go to Burke Rehabilitation Hospital in Westchester. The medical director at Cliffside had recommended it. Although I lived in Bethlehem, Pennsylvania, I'd had the stroke on my job in New York, so I wanted that facility in New York. I had heard it was one of the best.

By Tuesday no arrangements had been made. The social worker returned and explained that she was waiting on authorization from the insurance company. Meanwhile I was distributing my flowers and plants among the hospital staff, my friends, and sending some home with my husband.

Later on that afternoon the social worker came back to my room to inform me that I would be going to Burke Rehabilitation Hospital on Wednesday instead. I was looking forward to going so I could start my physical and occupational therapy and try to get back to normalcy as best as I could. That day was spent as usual with my many visitors. Vince was with me all day, only leaving for about two hours to take a rest in the apartment.

CHAPTER 4

Wednesday arrived at last, the day I was to go to Burke Rehabilitation Hospital. I was very excited. The nurses told me I had to have my medication and all my paperwork had to be completed before I left. The ambulette would be there at ten. That was the longest wait I had, but eventually the ambulette did come. Vince was there to help me. As an orderly wheeled me out of the hospital and into the ambulette, the driver checked to make sure my chair was properly secured.

As he placed the seat belt around me and snapped it into place, my mind suddenly went back to Cliffside Nursing Home. On many occasions I had said to the nursing assistant, "Please make sure the residents are secured safely. Please make sure to put on their seat belts." I never thought I would be in this position at this time of my life.

The ride to Westchester was surreal. *This is not me,* I kept thinking. I was Superwoman. I could do everything that was thrown at me in the office. If I didn't know how to do something,

I learned. I never said, "No, I cannot do it," or, "I don't know how to do it." Many times someone would say to me, "Yvonne, you are taking on too much," but I loved it. I really loved my job. My employers were great people to work with, and my working environment was wonderful. At no time did I feel that I did not want to go to work. I always said that there were not enough hours in the day. I really missed my job and was not ready to leave.

As we started our journey, I kept looking back at my husband following in his SUV. *What a tough break for him,* I thought. He had stopped working years prior to take care of his previous wife. He sold one of the two apartment buildings he owned in the Bronx so he could devote his time to her. He did that for more than fifteen years, until she died.

She did not have functioning kidneys, and he spent his life taking care of her, making sure she got to her many dialysis appointments and going to various hospitals in different states to get her on different kidney transplant lists. He devoted his life to her. That was why I admired him so much.

We met seven months after her death, and he was in a very depressed state. He was not ready to move on with his life, and I knew he was still in mourning. A year earlier my daughter and his son went to Las Vegas with some friends and got married quietly without any fanfare. They had decided to have a reception on their first wedding anniversary where they would invite all the family, that day was the first time we met. We spoke with each other at the reception and then started talking frequently on the telephone.

I knew he needed a friend to talk with, but I did not want to intrude. I wanted him to have his space, though everyone could see he was lonely. Meanwhile, I was not looking to get involved with anyone. My life was perfect as it was, or so I thought. My matchmaking daughter Jillian was pushing for the relationship; she was jumpstarting my last nerve.

I noticed Vince was hesitant to talk to me about his life, yet again I could see that he wanted to talk about his wife. I said to him, "You don't have to be afraid to talk to me about your wife. You can do that until the cows come home. That will not be a problem."

I encouraged him to talk about his wife because they had been happily married for thirtyfive years, and he was like a fish out of water without her.

Also, it was therapy for him. I did not want him to think it was going to get me upset or that I would shun him. He had a wonderful life before he ever knew I existed. He and his wife had a good marriage with lots of love. Also, I had a wonderful life and an excellent job, and I was not looking to change that in a hurry. I did what I wanted to do, when I wanted to do it, and that was great for me.

Although Vince invited me to his home, I wouldn't go. It just did not feel right to me. His neighbors would complement him when they saw us together, saying later that he had a special strut when he entered his building. I told him I would not visit his home until we'd known each other for a year and that he had to take me to his wife's grave first. I felt strongly about that. I needed to give his wife that respect, deep down though, I also did not want any commitment to any man at that time. I had been there and done that, and I wanted my freedom.

Now here was my husband following this ambulette after five years together and two years of marriage. Was it going to scare him off? Was he going to say, "I cannot go through this again"? Lots of crazy things were going through my mind. Although I tried to be brave, I knew I needed him. God had put him in my life at the right time, and I had almost blown it. Still, if he said to me he couldn't go through something like this again, I wouldn't fault him. Although I needed him more than ever now, I would have said okay and let him go.

I knew if it were the reverse and he was desperately ill, I would definitely stay with him and take care of him the best I could. He deserved that, but I just did not know how well he would be able to cope with another sick wife. As time proved, I was worrying needlessly. My husband became my anchor. He is such a positive man. He would look at me in the wheelchair and say, "You will be fine and recover fully."

I said to him one day, "You must have been very bad when you were younger, because you've had to look after not one but two sick wives. You really have to work very hard now to get to heaven." He laughed.

He knew my right side was completely paralyzed, but it did not faze him. Almost thirteen years my senior, he is as steady as a rock and he believes in family. He says to me that a man should protect his family. When people compliment him or say they admire him for taking care of me, he will reply, "What is there to admire? If I was the sick one, I would hope my wife would be there to take care of me. That is what marriage is about." I love this man.

While traveling to the rehabilitation hospital, I was admiring the scenery. It was a beautiful fall day. The trees were almost bare, and for the first time I was really aware of nature. I could see myself running in those multicolored leaves on the ground, rolling around in them. I suddenly realized that life is precious and it can be taken away from you in a minute. I had almost lost mine. Whew! It had taken an experience like this to make me realize how lucky I was. I decided I would do my best to help other stroke patients as soon as I was able to do volunteer work.

The ambulette turned into the driveway of Burke Rehabilitation Hospital. Wow! This place was great; it looked as though I was going to a resort. The long driveway to the main building looked serene and mysterious; all the trees were bare, but the place had an ambiance about it. In my mind I felt as though I was going on an adventure, not going to a hospital. There were many buildings on acres and acres of land; I thought it would be a very good place for rehabilitation. Well, this is it—time for my therapy to begin.

Burke Rehabilitation Hospital

I arrived at Burke Rehabilitation Hospital nine days after I had the stroke. As an orderly wheeled me upstairs, I saw some of the stroke patients going through their exercises sitting in their wheelchairs. Those patients were much older than I was. *I will be the youngest one here*, I thought. Although I was sixty, I did not feel that old. I decided to get rid of all of my mirrors when I got home. They had been lying to me for years. When I looked at myself, I saw a thirtyyearold woman, so enough was enough.

After seeing the patients exercising in the hallway, I knew rehab would be difficult at first but I would conquer it. I said under my breath, "Dear God, please help me."

Once I was in my room and was put in bed, I was desperate to go to the bathroom. I asked one of the nurses for a bedpan since I was unable to walk to go to the bathroom. After that, the nurses completed my admission by taking my vital signs and weight.

How ironic, I thought. When I was big and fat, I did not get a stroke. Now I'd lost more than fifty pounds and was a stroke patient. I had decided to lose the weight in the first place in order to control my blood sugar. I was keeping track of my blood pressure as well. I did not go on just any diet. My doctor had me on a particular one in which my weight loss was monitored.

I used to be a very large person with lots of health problems—diabetes, high blood pressure, and sleep apnea. My blood sugar was out of control, so my endocrinologist told me I had to lose weight. My stomach was too big, and I had to sleep with a CPAP machine. He put me on the Medifast diet. I had to have a shake or oatmeal in the morning, a candy bar midmorning, another shake for lunch and different snacks in the afternoon, and then for supper I had three to six ounces of chicken, turkey, or fish. It was very difficult for me. I never thought I could do it, but I did.

I was always a big eater, and what made it worse is that my husband loves to cook. I would smell his cooking and decide to cheat on my diet, but then I thought about my health. So I took it one day at a time. After two weeks I decided to quit. I'd had enough; I couldn't do it anymore. The receptionist at the doctor's office told me, "You might think that you are hungry, but you are not." What was she talking about? *I was hungry.*

However, Fran, my friend and colleague at work, straightened me out. "You can do it," she said, "and you are going to do it. Think of your health." She was so supportive but firm with me. I guess she was fed up with my whining, but being a former teacher, she knew how to deal with children (because I was really acting like a child). She encourages people in times of weakness. So I continued with my diet, strongly suggesting to my husband to please eat before I got home.

One year later I had lost fiftytwo pounds, and it was worth it. I looked good. I went from a women's size 18 to a size 10. I enjoyed getting a completely new wardrobe and showing off my new self. Now here I was, not using my CPAP machine anymore and with my medications reduced, but I had a stroke.

After I was settled in my bed, Vince came into the room. I was so glad to see him. We arranged for the television to be turned on by my bed, and then we just talked. He kept telling me everything was going to be all right. Finally it was time for him to leave as it was getting dark. He was unfamiliar with the winding Hutchinson Parkway; he had never been this far up the parkway before.

CHAPTER 5

When Vince left, a sudden wave of loneliness overtook me. *Why?* I thought. Vince had always been at the other hospital during the day and had left at night. Shortly after he left, a lovely nursing assistant came to my room. Smiling, she welcomed me to the facility and got me acquainted with everything. I couldn't hear a word she was saying because I was crying so hard. I suddenly missed my husband. I wasn't sure if it was the fact that he had to leave much earlier or if it was the distance from the hospital to our apartment, but I was a basket case.

Reality was upon me. I couldn't stop crying. It was as if my world had just collapsed. I had been so strong at the hospital. My husband was only ten minutes away, and he usually stayed until the announcement that visitors had to leave. Now he had to leave before it got dark because he couldn't see well at night and the road was unfamiliar to him. Since I'd had the stroke, my feeling was that I'd get up one day and I'd be fine. I had never spent so many days in a hospital before.

The nursing assistant asked if things were that bad. I did not want to listen to her. All I wanted was to go home with my husband. Although I had been excited to start my therapy, all common sense left me at that moment. I called my husband when I knew he was in the apartment and, still bawling my eyes out, told him to come back for me.

"I want to get out of here now. Come back and get me out."

I guess I had a moment of insanity. My poor husband was very upset. I could hear the stress in his voice. He told me he would come to get me the next day.

"No," I said. "Now."

I wanted him now. I wanted to sleep in his arms. I wanted him to come back for me now.

I know now what it means to have temporary insanity. All my logic went out the window at that time, and I was unable to stop crying. I wasn't behaving like myself. Something had abruptly taken over my mind. My faith hit the floor with a loud thud.

That night was very long. For some reason I wanted to go to the bathroom every hour all night long. I did not have an IV drip, and I did not consume much liquid that evening, only a cup of tea. All night I had to press the call bell so that someone could bring me that dreaded bedpan. I knew they were annoyed with me but were too gracious to say so. Finally I fell asleep only to be awakened by a nurse taking my vital signs. She then got me out of bed and propped me up in a wheelchair to get me washed and dressed.

After breakfast I had to wait for my weekly therapy schedule and to get a lap tray. The tray would keep me upright in the wheelchair and give me a place to put my right hand. Otherwise, it would just fall to the side of the chair and get entangled in the wheel. I was not upset that day, just waiting patiently to begin. Now I know a good cry was all I'd needed. Still, the crying I had done the night before was way out there. Deep down I might have been scared, or I had just needed to let out some pentup emotions. Whatever it was, I simply bound the spirit of fear and cast it out of my body in Jesus's name. (I wasn't too good with that either, but I spoke with authority.)

Sicknesses can really make you think, and you learn to lean even more on God.

My first therapy was speech. I had to endure many questions, writing exercises, and puzzles. The therapist probably saw my bewilderment. I wanted to know why I had to do this. Everything looked like it was geared toward young children. Also, I could speak and could do the puzzles. My problem was writing; I had to use my left hand, and that was very difficult. I thought I was wasting time. I needed to go do my physical and recreational therapy, not waste time with this.

The speech therapist told me a stroke can cause a person to lose control of the muscles in her mouth and throat, making it difficult to talk, swallow, or eat. That can cause slurred speech. She also told me a stroke victim could have difficulty speaking or understanding speech, reading, or writing. By having speech, physical, and occupational therapy all together, my skills would improve.

These exercises might seem menial, she said, but they provided information on a patient's condition and how the brain was healing. While giving me all these exercises to do, she also told me that many people who have had a stroke can sustain some memory loss and difficulty thinking and understanding simple instructions. She then gave me the swallowing evaluation with a thickened liquid. Half an hour later, the nurse came to wheel me to the physical therapy department.

The daytoday routine seem mundane at first, but I was ready for my workout. It was so difficult at first I thought I was going to collapse, but nothing was going to beat me. I had physical and occupational therapy twice a day, Monday through Friday, and once on Saturday. Speech therapy was only once a day Monday through Friday.

That first day was grueling. The therapy was a real workout for me. I used to go to Bally's gym and spend two hours working out. Now they had me on a bike for five minutes and I felt as though I'd run a marathon. My right foot would not stay on the bike pedal, so the therapist strapped it on.

After the bike the therapist put on a foot brace. She got me standing, she and an aide holding me upright, and tried to get me to use a walker so that I could take a few steps. They also had to use a Velcro strap around my right hand because it could not grip or even stay on the walker. Still I thought I was doing well. Some of the patients couldn't get out of bed. *God is good,* I told myself. Soon I wouldn't need all of this. I would do it on my own.

I think I had the best therapist there. Her name was Kerry. She was so committed to her patients, although all the therapists were good and dedicated. Still, I was glad Kerry was my therapist.

When I returned to my room, I felt exhausted. That's when Vince came, followed by the kitchen staff with my supper. Vince saw me struggling with the food and offered to feed me. I gladly accepted. All that I wanted to do was sleep. He said, with a smirk on his face, "I am here to take you home. Do you still want to go home?"

"Have you gone and lost your mind?" I asked. "Were you really going to take me home? I'm fine now."

"I was just humoring you, honey, because you were driving me up a wall last night. I did not sleep well last night, so I had to take a drink."

I laughed because everything makes him take a drink. I asked if that was why he had called me at four o'clock that morning. I had vaguely heard the phone ringing but had not recognized what it was. When it was time for him to leave, I was happy because I couldn't concentrate and conversation was becoming difficult. I was extremely exhausted.

After he left, I collapsed in bed. I hazily heard the kitchen aide remove the tray as I drifted off to a deep sleep. I was rudely awakened by a nurse's aide.

"Yvonne," she said with a happy smile, "tonight I'm going to give you a shower."

What? I told her in no uncertain terms, "Please do not take God out of your thoughts and touch me tonight." I was unable to move from all that therapy. I went back to sleep immediately and slept like a baby, except for the two times I needed to go to the bathroom.

The routine the next morning was the same as the day before. I was woken up by the aide who helped me wash and dress, and then Rachel, the occupational therapist, had to teach me how to use the toothbrush with my left hand. Since I was right handed, it was extremely difficult. I had to place the toothbrush on the sink, put the toothpaste under my right arm (which was completely paralyzed), use my left hand to unscrew the cap, and then take the toothpaste in my left hand and squeeze it out onto the toothbrush. I then had to reverse the procedure to put the cap back on the toothpaste.

After that, I had to learn how to dress myself with only my left hand. I hooked my bra while sitting, put my right arm in first and then my good arm, got it over my head, and struggled to get it right. I had to have lots of help at first, but soon I was able to dress myself with ease. This made me realize how difficult it is for some people to do this every day. I really have great respect for the therapists for all their hard work and dedication. They make it look so easy.

One day the doctor came to see me and ordered me some pills that I was not familiar with. He tried to explain, saying that when a person has a stroke, he or she sometimes has difficulty controlling his or her emotions, which can cause depression.

"Well, that's not me," I said. "I am not depressed."

"Let's call this your happy pill," he said.

"I am very happy at this moment. Haven't you noticed? If I get any happier, the men in white coats will definitely take me away."

He laughed and said that some studies had found this medication helped the brain heal. I'm not sure if he was yanking my chain, but I started taking the medication—anything to heal the brain. But as soon as I left the rehabilitation hospital, I discontinued taking those pills.

Each day the nurse came around with pain medication. I refused to take it because I had no pain in my body. Why were they always bringing me painkillers? I didn't know that I was going to have pain much later, and with such ferocity. One of my aides told me she'd known one patient with so much pain that she was unable to sleep at night. I just thought I was lucky.

At eight in the morning I got my medications and an injection in my stomach, that medication left my stomach a bluishpurple. Then I had my breakfast and was ready for speech therapy at nine. The nurse came for me and took me to the speech therapist's office. My therapist was lovely. (I've forgotten her name.) She gave me things to read and assessed how much my brain was affected. I was very alert. The only sign of the stroke was my slightly twisted mouth, which was not even noticeable because I always had my nutmeg in my mouth.

She wanted to know how often I put the nutmeg in my mouth because she was afraid I would swallow it. She again explained to me that when people suffered from a stroke, their swallowing reflexes were not that good and they could choke easily. I told her I always kept the nutmeg in, but at night I removed it.

Even before the stroke I usually swallowed liquids slowly because I always cough. Having the nutmeg in my mouth made no difference. During the daytime I only took it out to eat and brush my teeth. I would not recommend anyone drinking or sleeping with a nutmeg in his or her mouth. I told the therapist it was a Caribbean thing, to straighten out your mouth when you have a stroke.

She decided to research the nutmeg on the Internet. She found an article and was fascinated by what she learned. She wanted to know where anyone could buy whole nutmegs in the United States. I told her she could get them anywhere that there is a large West Indian population, at fruitandvegetable stores, and even at some supermarkets.

Word got around the hospital about the nutmeg, and both patients and their visitors wanted to know about the nutmeg and where to obtain it. Soon after my stroke, someone had taken a picture of my twisted mouth with my phone. People who saw that picture taken before I used the nutmeg and then saw me after using it were amazed.

Sometimes I became frustrated, after my swallowing evaluation and speech therapy five days a week. I had to do those puzzles and write with my left hand, which was extremely difficult. Then the nurses would take me to occupational therapy. After that hour, next was physical therapy, which was still difficult for me. I had lunch at one o'clock, and then back I went to physical therapy at two o'clock, and then from there to occupational therapy for another hour.

One time occupational therapy was in the corridor where I had seen the patients on my first day. We were stretching, throwing a ball to each other, and doing different rangeofmotion exercises when I saw a younger man coming to join our group. My curiosity was piqued. Surely he was much too young to have had a stroke. I was informed by another patient that he was a doctor who also had a stroke.

I had never known young people got strokes. But my occupational therapist had had a stroke and she was in her thirties, and now this doctor. I learned later on he was only fortynine.

CHAPTER 6

One day when I was finished with the occupational therapy and it was time to wind down before supper, a recreational therapist came to get me involved in games and movies, and I was not interested. However, a counselor invited us to a meeting downstairs for all the new patients, and I went to that. Her duty was to let us know about strokes and how it had changed our lives. We were told that we had a higher risk of getting another stroke within five years. That was not reassuring, but I knew that was not for me. I would *never* have another stroke. She also told us we would not be able to drive again in New York until we took another driving test.

My mother had had three strokes, and I had never fully understood what she was going through because she never complained. I know now that I have to break the cycle, so I declare and believe that this stroke was the last and it ended with me. Being disabled is a lifechanging thing. You have to adjust to the difficult task ahead, but you can do it. Sometimes you have some crazy ideas and feelings in your head, but you soon get over them.

I had my computer and iPad to keep me occupied, so after therapy I went to my room and read my Bible, refusing to focus on what was mentioned in the meeting.

On another day a lovely lady named Diane came to my room to talk about a research study Burke Rehab was conducting. She wanted to know if I would be interested in being a subject in the study. She explain that there were no side effects, and it would help the brain to heal faster.

That phrase again, I thought. *It helps the brain to heal.*

I told her I would get back to her the next day and called a few people, including the nursing director from Cliffside. Everyone said it wouldn't hurt, so I decided I would try any—and everything that would get me back on my feet sooner rather than later. So I informed Diane that I would participate in the study. After that, every morning the night nurse woke me at five to take five tiny pills. This went on for about three to four weeks.

I realize now that it is very important to start your therapy immediately after a stroke. It helps the brain to begin working again. I will not say it's easy because it is not. At the time of the therapy, my right hand was completely paralyzed, and the only thing I could have done was to massage it with my left hand. There was absolutely no movement. I was lucky, because I always had sensation on my right side, but I was unable to move both my arm and leg.

I had a dropped foot, so the doctor ordered a foot splint to help me walk. My attending doctor, Dr. Mary, told me to talk to my hand. I laughed because I thought that if someone saw me talking to my hand, they might have me carted away to the loony bin. I must stress, however, that *talking to the hand works*. Don't ask me how, but a neurologist can explain it to you. I include my paralyzed hand in everything I do.

So I would talk to the hand, and one day I saw a slight twinge of the thumb. Well, you would have thought I had just won the lottery. I called everyone around to see it. They stared at my hand and looked at each other, laughing at my enthusiasm and not seeing anything, but I saw it. The most important thing was *I* saw it. No matter how tired, depressed, or in pain you are, *do not refuse your therapy*. And always talk to your affected limbs.

One day as I sat talking to my hand, my mind drifted to the residents at Cliffside, wondering if this serene feelings I had, was what they had felt. I used to talk to them and loved it when they smiled. When there was an entertainer at the facility, I would go off to the dining room and dance for the residents and join in the entertainment. As I am from the Caribbean, the residents always called out to me to dance to the soca music. We had lots of fun dancing to soca and reggae. It really made me happy to see their smiling faces.

Cliffside is a very nice place to live and work. The only reason I was at Burke was because the doctor had told me I needed to be in an acutecare facility and Cliffside is a subacute facility. I knew it wouldn't be long before I was dancing like I once had before the stroke.

For a while they had to tie my foot to one of the pedals in order for me to pedal a bike; I did this until I did not need my foot to be tied anymore. My time on the machine reached fifteen minutes. That was a milestone for me. Then I wanted to advance to another level because my leg was getting stronger.

Other patients would squeeze a rubber ball to strengthen their hands. I did not have one because I was unable to make a fist, so I continued to talk to the hand. You should have seen me, massaging the hand and talking away. I was still unable to squeeze even a piece of sponge, so I kept talking to the hand. About the third week of my therapy I had slight movement in my index finger. Everyone knew they had to stare at it for a while before they would see any movement. Sometimes my visitors would say it was in my head, but Vince always said, "Yes, dear, it moved." I know that he did not really see it, but he was giving me encouragement. I saw it, though, and that was the most important thing.

There was an Irish patient who went to therapy at the same time as I did. He made me laugh every day. If his wife was visiting, he would stay in his room with her. But as soon as she left, he would visit my room, telling Vince and me jokes. He had a great sense of humor. Sometimes we laughed really loud and were unable to control our laughter, so the nurses would come in to see what was going on. I swear, that man could have had his own show. When a therapist would ask us if we needed a drink of water, he would always say, "All I want is a beer." He broke up the monotony of the daily routine, making my stay easier and time go by more quickly.

Previous patients would come to give us pep talks and show us how they were getting along. One evening we all gathered, waiting for a former stroke patient to come speak to us, and in walked a lovely blonde in high heels. I wondered if she was accompanying the former patient. When she stated that she was a former patient and had had two strokes, we all gasped. She showed no sign ever having had a stroke, which really boosted my morale. I was captivated by her and hung on to her every word.

Suddenly one of the patients started to curse God. I was stunned. She kept repeating that she had been a good person all her life, and there were many murderers, rapists, and thieves out there who should have had a stroke, but God had given it to her instead. All of the other patients got angry at her. It became difficult for her to stay, so she left the room. She was a very bitter lady. I was also disgusted with her, but later on I realized she had lost her faith and had no hope. I prayed for her, but I never saw her again. No matter how dismal the circumstances may look, you must never give up. Keep your faith.

CHAPTER 7

About three weeks after I had the stroke, while sitting in my room, I started flipping through the television channels and stopped when I saw a woman preacher. I had never heard of her before; I only listened to Joel Osteen because he is a different kind of preacher from other television preachers. He motivates me and makes me look at things differently than I otherwise would.

It was as if this woman was talking to me. The things she was saying sounded familiar, so I instantly changed the channel. I had partnered with Joel Osteen; that's why he was the only person I would watch. I was not religious; I just loved to watch him because he was so positive. Even if I am down, after hearing his jokes and message, my spirits will soar to the highest height.

So I continued flipping again, but without realizing it, I was back on that same channel. There she was again, talking about herself and all she had gone through. I could not believe what I was hearing. She sounded real and not like preachers who are quick to judge and condemn. I just listened to her. She said her name was Joyce Myers.

From that day on I had to find her on whatever channel she was on. I even have Vince listen to her. I had never heard of Joyce Myers before, and now I always listen to her message. At first, I felt as if I was being dishonest to Joel, but there were similarities with their messages. I have many of Joyce Myers's books, but still I start my Sundays with Joel Osteen.

When I am alone, I sometimes assess my life because things that were important to me are no longer important. I pray and just thank God for his blessings and for the healing that has taken place in my body. I've learned not to focus on the symptoms but to exercise my faith and belief. Ask for anything in Jesus's name, and it is done. I really believe and continue to thank God, because I know that my God has healed me.

I was making good progress. Everyone said so, including Dr. Mary. I was able to dress myself after many tries, and I was able to wash and take care of myself. Hygiene was very important to me, and although taking care of myself was not easy, I was determined to master the task, and I did.

Rachel, my occupational therapist, was very thorough. When she told me about the stroke she'd had a few years earlier and what she had done to get to this point in her life, I was even more determined to heal. There was no sign that she'd ever had a stroke. I admired her and knew I would make it. If she could do it, so could I. It was torture at first to do everything with my left hand, but I managed to get along.

Rachel had me sort out my medications. That was one of the things I took for granted. I wondered why I was doing such menial things. I told her I could read, but then I realized it was very important to practice. From then on I did not question why. I learned to fold clothes and to transfer from a chair to the bath.

Kerry, my physical therapist, had to be comfortable with me using the walker before she would let me keep one in my room. Eventually she did, and I was elated. I had to use the wheelchair only at night. I started going to therapy on my own. That was a major achievement for me.

I spent Thanksgiving at the rehab center with my children, grandchildren, sister, and other friends. We all gathered downstairs where my family had decorated tables with flowers and a massive amount of food. My sister told me she'd been up all night cooking. There were about fifteen of us, and we had a wonderful time. My grandchildren had fun pushing me around in the wheelchair.

During the meal, while everyone was joking and laughing with one another, my sister told me about that first night of the stroke, when she heard me babbling over the phone. She demonstrated the sound, and we all had a good laugh. She said she had been unable to stop crying. She called a friend, still crying, and her friend tried hard to console her. She told me that considering the way I had sounded then and how my recovery was going now, she had to tell her church members about my progress. They were all praying for me.

After everyone had left that evening, Vince helped me get changed into my nightclothes, and then I collapsed in bed. He did not have to worry about driving in the dark, so his son took him home after he helped me into bed.

As I said before, I think I had the best physical therapist. Kerry was well liked at the hospital. She was very focused on her job and always had patience with me. One thing that embarrassed me was that since I had the stroke, I was unable to hold in my gas. It came out anytime, anywhere, and most of the time during therapy.

There was nothing I could do about it, so I suffered in silence with great embarrassment. She would say, "Don't worry about it, it's natural." Well, it was not natural for me, but it just continued. She gave me lots of different exercises. I thought some of them were useless, but after doing them I realized that each and every one was vital and essential for my recovery. No matter how childish an exercise looks, it is geared toward aiding your body or stimulating some function in the brain.

Please Do Not Feel Sorry for Yourself, but Stay Positive and Focused

I broke down that first night and felt sorry for myself, but not again. Even if you do not feel like doing anything, don't let selfpity take over. If you do not push through the pain, you *will* get worse. Do what you can, don't overdo it, and always do your therapy. Keep a rubber ball handy so you can use it intermittently to strengthen your muscles. Keep the affected hand occupied with the ball. Even if you have visitors, keep that ball handy and just squeeze it.

When I left the rehab center, I did not have any home help. I had only Vince to rely on. I knew that was quite a bit of responsibility for him, and his hands were going to be full just looking after me. He rushed to the pharmacy to get my medications and then was so attentive to me. My meals were always on time. He fussed over me at night, and always helped me along. I know I can never repay him for all he has done for me. I am a very lucky woman, and I cannot and will not take that for granted.

Six weeks into my recovery, when I was still unable to return to work, I got that dreaded letter of termination from my job. It was one of the saddest days of my life. Although I knew it was only business and not personal, and that it had to be done because they had to fill my position, it still was not easy.

One weekend Vince's niece came for a visit. She is exactly like me, loving our Trinidad carnival and soca music. We started to play the latest soca music, and she got up to dance. I did not want to be outdone, so I got up, holding on to my cane, and started to dance as well. Although I was unsteady on my feet, I was having a good time. I was coming back to my old self.

Vince got so scared seeing me dancing, he said in a loud voice, "If you fall, I am done. You can stick me with a fork and turn me over." That is another of his sayings. We paid no attention to him and just continued dancing. That weekend visit was very enjoyable.

When I went to visit my friends at Cliffside, I refused to use the walker. I had one of my colleagues come to the car so I could hold on to her hand as I walked inside. I just did not want the employees to see me with a walker; it was my pride again. Some of the residents at the home used walkers. Everyone was so happy to see me and all the progress I'd made. The Director's office got very crowded as the incoming evening staff and outgoing day staff stopped in.

There were lots of laughter and hugs. It felt nice to be back, even if it was for such a short time. I stayed for about three hours, but I finally had to leave. That was a sad moment for me.

Another time my daughter came from Maryland and suggested we walk a few feet outside.

"You've got to be crazy," I said. "The neighbors will see me. I am not going out there with a leg brace and using a walker."

That pride raised its ugly head again.

I soon got out of that foolishness, because the only thing I should have pride in now is how well I have done and all the improvements I've made. I finally went out with my leg brace and walker to the community center. I became a member and started doing various activities, which I continue to do to this day. Each day I look at the outdoor running track and know it is only a matter of time before I will be running around it; but for now I use the inside track. I walk for a mile and then go on the treadmill. Using a very slow setting, I stay on it for a half hour.

CHAPTER 8

If you are a family member or a caregiver, or know anyone who's had a stroke, and they cannot do the exercises and you can help them, please do so. If nothing is done, their limbs will atrophy. It is so rewarding when you see the stages someone goes through, from unable to move to complete recovery.

If you've had a stroke and are having difficulty opening your hand, ask your therapist for a splint to put on your hand at night. This helps the fingers stay outstretched. Another thing that can be very painful for a stroke victim is yawning. For some reason everything on the affected side moves. Your fingers clench like claws, and your toes stretch. Sometimes you have to unclench your fingers with your other hand or ask someone to open it for you. If it cannot open, don't force it. Your physical therapist will recommend something for you to keep in your hand.

I learned that if you do not have feeling in the affected arm or leg, there will be no pain. I want feeling, so I thank God every night and day for my pains. Although it can be excessive, I still thank him because the pain tells me I am healing.

A therapist once told me that the legs heal faster because the brain has no choice but to try to recover the damaged areas, and you are constantly using your legs to walk. The arms are the most difficult to heal, as they are the farthest from the brain. I did not understand that concept, so I said to her that the legs appear to be farther. She explained that although the legs are further from the brain, we have to use our legs to walk and this helps the affected part of the brain to work. Therefore, it is a pity we don't use our hands to walk on also. I thought that I should walk on my hands as some sort of exercise. Then I said to myself, *Self, if I am on the floor. Who is going to get me up? And furthermore, there is no way I could get down on the floor.* So I decided against it.

Occasionally I fell, but it was because I was trying to do things that I wasn't ready to do. That did not faze me. I just tried to be much more careful whenever I attempted to do something.

I cannot stress it enough—always try to do any kind of therapy. If your insurance won't pay for it anymore and you cannot afford it on your own, join a community center or a YMCA. You can walk around the track or do exercises in the pool, which is what I did. Doing this will be very beneficial.

My goal is still to volunteer with stroke patients as soon as I am able to do so. I know I have something to offer and can help to motivate them. I look at myself and realize it is now a year and a half since I had the stroke, and it is amazing what I can do. I can walk with a cane, shower and dress myself, and take care of all of my personal hygiene. I vacuum the bedrooms sometimes (which takes forever), and every day I make the bed. Also, I've done the laundry and folded the clothes, but I need help folding the sheets. I do anything I can that will help me get back to my regular routine.

Many people still comment on my progress, stating that I do not look as though I ever had a stroke. Although I look that way, my limbs are still weak and I will stumble at times. Still, that does not deter my determination to recover completely and get on with my life. Sometimes I can walk without using my cane in the house.

One year and two months after the stroke, I had decided that I needed to work but was unable to do so. Who was going to employ me at this stage? I would be a liability to any company. Also, I am over sixty, I've had a stroke and still need therapy, and. I get exhausted easily and have to rest regularly.

I take keepfit classes at the community center, and most of the time I do my exercises while sitting in a chair. It is so much fun. The women there are so friendly and helpful, and I am making lots of friends. After the keepfit classes I usually take the stairs instead of the elevator. Climbing stairs is also therapy for me.

Some of the exercises are difficult for me, but that is not a problem. The instructor encourages me when I make the effort, but she will tell me not to overdo it, just to do what I can. I think the center is very lucky to have Kathy as an instructor. All the ladies love her, and she shows concern for people like me who are much slower. Whenever another instructor is doing the class, I do not attend. This is not to say the other instructors aren't good, I am just more comfortable with Kathy. On Wednesday she teaches yoga. I love that class as well because all the stretches are exactly what my right arm need.

My husband had me laughing so hard after one of the classes—as I said before, he should have been a comedian. He said, "Baby, you should have seen yourself from behind," and his impression of me had us laughing uncontrollably. It was a sight to behold; he was doing all sorts of contortions with his body. He then told me he knew I was trying my best and that's what counted. "So do not give up, baby. Keep trying."

When I see my husband walking out of the house with his clothes looking as though they just came out of a basket with crumpled clothes, it saddens me. So I am now going to iron his clothes, since we cannot afford to take everything to the cleaners. That is also therapy for my hand.

A year after I had the stroke, I got a call from Diane at Burke Rehabilitation Hospital. I was astonished that they still knew who I was. She was the doctor's assistant who had enrolled me in the study while I was a patient there. They wanted me to be in another one, she said, mentioning that I was one of her favorite patients there at that time.

She told me that everyone had admired my determination and persistence when I was there. So this time it was an approved drug already being given to people with multiple sclerosis.

They were trying it out on patients who had a stroke over six months. They were trying to prove it helped the patients' limbs move better and improved their walking. If the studies indicated that, they could get the medication approved for stroke patients. I considered that I had fond memories of that facility and, as I said to my husband, I was all for anything that could heal me faster. He agreed.

So for more than a month we made the trip to New York every week. It was great to see other former patients there in the hospital's outpatient clinic having followup visits with their doctor. It may have been all in my head, but at the end of the study I thought my walking was much better. All the different tests I did with the physical therapist showed significant improvement. She was impressed.

When it was over, I was sad to leave the study, but a few months later I received a letter with a check. It was a stipend for my travels. Although I did not know they would give me money and I had not been looking for any, it was a nice surprise.

We took a twoweek vacation to Florida after the study, deciding to take the train from Virginia so we could take our vehicle without having to drive. I felt like a kid again. It has been years since I'd been on a train. I was amazed by how easy it was to get around. The two resorts where we stayed in Florida were very accommodating to disabled patrons. They had power chairs for me to get around.

We went to Orlando and St. Petersburg, and although I was moving slowly and got tired easily, I had a wonderful time. The thing that impressed me the most was that I actually did all our packing and unpacking by myself. That was a major achievement for me. I can see the light at the end of the tunnel.

All of my adult life I have worked, so you can imagine being at home had me stircrazy. I kept myself busy by going to the center and accompanying my husband to the supermarket. On one occasion we went to do some grocery shopping with my granddaughter Tsashai. I did not realize that an employee at the store used to flirt with Vince and always assisted him when he was looking for a particular product. While shopping I got very tired and decided that I would wait for Vince and Tsashai near the checkout counters.

After waiting for what seemed like an eternity, I saw them in a checkout line closer to the door. When Vince was finished, he beckoned to me to come and meet them, but then suddenly he ran out of the supermarket with my granddaughter in tow. That seemed odd to me, because anyone who knows him understands that he wouldn't leave me behind. He will always be there to hold my hand.

When I got outside, he was waiting in the vehicle. He came around to help me get in. I asked him what that was all about. Tsashai said, "I told him to wait for Mimi." Vince just said that we had to go. He told me that since it was raining, he had wanted to get the car so that I wouldn't get wet.

"Yeah, right," I said.

Later on he told me, laughing, that when he beckoned me to join them, the woman who worked there thought he was gesturing to her. Both of us started walking toward him at the same time, so he ran. Ah! You should have seen his face, so proud that women still think he's gorgeous—which he is. Everyone who knows us knows he wouldn't stray. He is really a devoted husband. Still, it inflated his ego, and I was happy for him that he still has it. I can only imagine what he had been saying to that woman when he was shopping alone.

So I can be prepared when the time comes for me to return to a job, I am going to take an online class. I can only type with one finger at the moment, and my filing ability has been greatly reduced, which is a problem. Also, I feel as though I'm always running a marathon whenever I try to do any work task. I get so exhausted, but I am not letting that keep me down. I did not realize what the stroke was going to take out of me, but I am enduring it. Things are really getting better. Time goes by slowly, but I am doing it.

I was told that being a stroke patient, my recovery will require continuous exercising, so I do not neglect it. Remember, a stroke can happen to anyone, not just the elderly as I had thought. So if you are at a high risk, check in frequently with your doctor and monitor yourself. You hold the key to your recovery: stay positive and believe. Give thanks for the little things in life. Take small steps at a time and persevere at whatever you do. Never give up.

My mother taught me years ago to help as many people as I could when I was on my way up in life, because if I happen to fall, they are the same people I will meet on my way down. All of my life I have tried to live by that motto.

I was denied disability benefits because, as social security put it, I am not disabled enough; I am not sure how much more disabled I have to be. I cannot completely use my hand, cannot walk without an assistive device, am unsteady on my feet, and will sometimes fall when I push myself to walk without a cane. I have appealed the decision, so at the moment I am waiting to go to court. As I mentioned before, if Vince weren't in my life, I really do not know what I would have done.

I cannot wait to volunteer to help stroke patients. When I can, I will be out the door as fast as I can. That day cannot come soon enough. I know it will give me such joy to help someone.

Remember, words are powerful. Whatever you say to the universe happens. I used to say that I would love to stay home for a few months to enjoy my new house. Now I have. I always wished I was left handed. Now I am. So always speak positive words about your life. I am living proof that it works.

I always count my blessings for what I can do and don't dwell on what I cannot do. So before I go to bed, I always visualize myself getting into my car and driving to the mall to do my shopping. Then I say I am blessed, I am strong, I am healthy, and I am healed. After that I usually cover myself, my family, and friends with the word.

The light of God surrounds me, the love of God enfolds me,
the power of God protects me.
Praise God, amen.

www.ingramcontent.com/pod-product-compliance
Lightning Source LLC
Chambersburg PA
CBHW050428290526
45786CB00003B/1441
* 9 7 8 1 4 9 0 7 1 4 7 7 6 *